365 ways to

# ENERGIZE

mind, body & soul

# 365 ways to

# ENERGIZE
## mind, body & soul

STEPHANIE TOURLES

STOREY BOOKS

Schoolhouse Road
Pownal, VT 05261

*The mission of Storey Communications is to serve our customers by publishing practical information that encourages personal independence in harmony with the environment.*

Edited by Deborah Balmuth and Karen Levy
Cover and text design by Carol Jessop
Book layout by Susan Bernier
Production Assistance by Deb Daly
Copyright © 2000 by Stephanie Tourles

Storey books are available for special premium and promotional uses and for customized editions. For further information, please call Storey's Custom Publishing Department at 800-793-9396.

Printed in the United States by Command Web
10 9 8 7 6 5 4 3 2

### Library of Congress Cataloging-in-Publication Data

Tourles, Stephanie L., 1962-
 365 ways to energize mind, body & soul / Stephanie Tourles.
 p. cm.
 ISBN 1-58017-3314 (alk. paper)
 1. Conduct of life. 2. Vitality. I. title: Three hundred sixty-five ways to energize mind, body & soul. II. Title.
BF637.C5 T68 2000
158.1′28—dc21

00-057395

# Dedication

To my precious William, I dedicate this book. You're truly my soul mate, my destined partner, and the love of my life. This year on August 25th we celebrate our 10th wedding anniversary. I can't believe how fast the years have passed, and I long for a lifetime of continued joy, laughter, and love with you, my darling. You've made my wildest dreams come true!

# Acknowledgments

To my dear editor, Deborah Balmuth: You inspire me to dig deep within and gently push me to realize that what I deemed impossible is indeed possible. Your support, combined with that of my husband Bill, enables me to accomplish anything with success and pride . . . and speed! Also, thanks to all of you who shared your tried and true methods of energy enhancement. I truly appreciate your inspiration.

# Introduction

**A**RE YOU IN THE THROES OF A PERSONAL ENERGY CRISIS? If so, you're not alone. Health practitioners report that fatigue, in its many forms, is the most common complaint heard from patients today.

Energy...what exactly is it? Most cultures have a name for it — *pneuma* in Greek, *neshamah* in Hebrew, *spiritus* in Latin, *qi* in Chinese, *prana* in Sanskrit, *ki* in Japanese — to refer to mental, physical, and spiritual life energy.

Although you can't physically hold it in your hands, you can see the sun's energy as light, feel it as warmth, and see evidence of it in the life around you. You can hear the invisible energy of thunder during a rainstorm and see purple bolts of lightning through the clouds. The stimulating effects of a nutritious diet can make you more aware of your strength and stamina.

Positive mental energy, too, can be transmitted through a kind word or a thoughtful gesture. Healing energy is conveyed through laying on of hands, Reiki, touch therapy, massage, or simple human contact. Energy can come in the form of inspiration, prayer, meditation, and exercise, as well as from time spent alone, in nature, and with family and friends.

Energy is vital. Energy is power. Along with oxygen and water, we need energy in order to survive and thrive. No matter how much we already have, we can always use more. We need large amounts of energy to get through our hectic schedules and deal with the demands of modern life; sadly, most of us don't have nearly enough of this precious resource. It's an elusive, mysterious force that courses through our being.

We know when we have it, and we know when it's flagging.

I hope these energizing tips will help guide you toward recharging your physical body, restoring your spirit, and revitalizing your mental capacities. May you recapture your zest for life, your happiness, your wholeness, and your physical stamina.

*Blessings of Abundant Energy*
*to You and Yours,*
Stephanie Tourles

# Bath Therapy

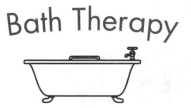

A warm, luxuriant bath is the ultimate way to boost your circulation and balance your energy flow. Pour a tall glass of your favorite beverage, close the door, turn the lights down, put on some background music, light a candle and perhaps some incense, and step in. Feel yourself melt into a pool of pleasure.

Keep a diet diary for a week and write down everything you eat. If your **PROTEIN** intake is less than 20–30 percent of your daily calories, you may feel fatigued. Add a few servings of organic eggs, lean poultry, beef, wild game, fish, whole grains, and beans to your weekly menu.

# AROMA THERAPY

For a quick energy boost,
keep a bottle of peppermint, cypress, eucalyptus,
spearmint, or geranium essential oil handy.
Place a few drops on a tissue and inhale deeply.

# Drink Up

Your brain's **weight** is more than 70 percent water. If this proportion drops below a certain point, you'll feel tired and headachy. Drink **eight glasses of water daily** — more if you're active or if it's hot. Coffee, black tea, and soft drinks don't count. They're diuretics, forcing your kidneys to excrete precious fluid from your body.

# Believe in yourself

and feel confident
that you can
**achieve anything**
you set your
mind to.

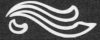

"Live each season
as it passes;
breathe the air,
drink the drink,
taste the fruit,
and resign yourself
to the influences
of each."

Henry David Thoreau

Midafternoon **ENERGY** slumps are often caused by low blood sugar. Be sure to eat a balanced lunch of lean protein, such as seafood, tofu, tempeh, or chicken, and a complex carbohydrate, such as whole grain bread, tabouli, beans, rice, or potatoes. A pat of butter or olive oil slows digestion, keeping blood sugar **STABLE** for several hours.

**FOLLOW** your heart without asking whether it's **OKAY** to do so.

Avoid eating turkey for lunch. It contains tryptophan, which can cause drowsiness.

"This is the true joy in life, the being used for a purpose recognized by yourself as a mighty one."

George Bernard Shaw

# Hit the Hay

Did you know that constant sleep deprivation
can depress your immune system? We try to
pack so much activity into our daily lives that
inadequate sleep has hit epidemic levels. Sooner
or later you'll pay the price with how you feel,
think, and look. Sleep is the best-kept beauty
and energy secret around.

Residents in nursing homes love to **TALK,** hold your hand, and relate their life stories. Listening to someone decades older than you can also be a fascinating lesson in **HISTORY.** Take the time to sit and chat for a while and you could make someone very **HAPPY.**

# Have Your Blood Tested

B-vitamin or iron deficiency can lead to an inadequate amount of oxygen in your blood, making you feel lethargic. Even if you think you're eating a healthy diet, you may not be getting enough of these essential nutrients, especially if you're a vegan (strict vegetarian) and/or premenopausal. If a blood test shows a deficiency, follow your doctor's orders by adjusting your diet accordingly. Your energy should soon return.

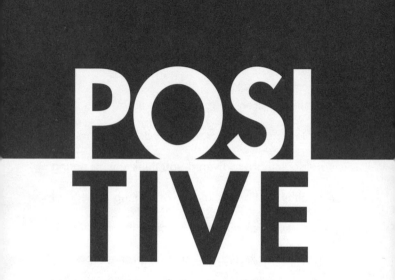

# POSI TIVE

Negative emotions drain your enthusiasm and zest for life. A positive attitude is refreshing and contagious. Surround yourself with people who are happy and have a strong sense of purpose.

# Put an end
to a bad
relationship.

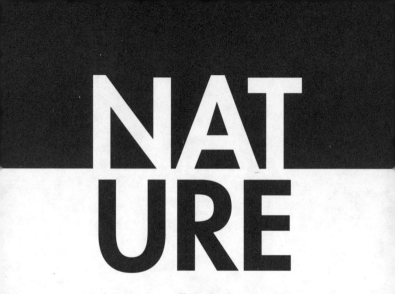

# NATURE

Mother Nature offers the best medicine
for your soul.

# Eat a Light Lunch

Loading up at lunch can leave you feeling tired, especially if you've eaten a carbohydrate-heavy meal of pasta, rice and beans, or bread. Eat a light or moderate lunch and you'll have more energy in the afternoon.

"Spread love everywhere you go: first of all in your own house."

MOTHER TERESA

# Smooth and Fruity Energy Shake

*Start your day with this high-protein, mineral-rich breakfast shake.*

### MAKES 2 SERVINGS

- 1 cup calcium-fortified, low-fat plain soy milk
- 1 cup orange juice
- 1 cup raspberries, peaches, strawberries, or pears
- ½ cup calcium-fortified soft tofu
- 1 banana
- 1 scoop soy protein powder
- 1 tablespoon wheat bran or oat bran

Combine all ingredients in a blender and whiz until smooth. Drink immediately.

# GREEN TEA

This earthy, natural energizer
is rich in antioxidants and has only one-fifth
the caffeine of black tea, so it won't make you
jittery or stain your teeth.

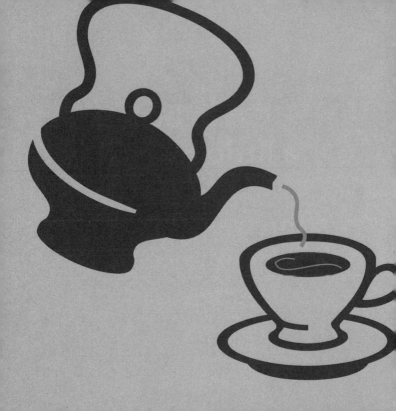

Go to bed
a little earlier.
It's better to get
some restful sleep
than watch
television.

# For the Birds

Take some bread, crackers, or sunflower seeds to the park to spend some time with your feathered friends. Marvel at the perfection of their feathers and listen to their variety of songs, squawks, and chirps. Notice how light they are on their feet.

Then let your energy take flight.

Update your look with a new **HAIRCUT,** makeup colors, or beard or mustache trim.

"Take a music bath
once or twice
a week for a few
seasons and you
will find that
it is to the soul
what the water bath
is to the body."

Oliver Wendell Holmes

# Breathe!

Try this exercise to help you refocus your energy:

* Stand with your feet shoulder-width apart and place your palms on your lower abdomen.

* Close your eyes and slowly inhale through your nose, gradually expanding your diaphragm. If you're breathing correctly, you will feel your hands move outward.

* Hold for a count of five, then exhale slowly through your mouth.

* Repeat 10 times.

Even if you're having a bad day, try to find at least one good thing that will bring a **SMILE** to your face. It takes more energy to frown, and the act of smiling will boost your energy.

"Those who dare and dare greatly are those who achieve."

Anonymous

# Wake Up!

Need a bit of afternoon stimulation? Falling asleep after lunch? A shot of oxygen is what you need. Perform this exercise to pump more of this life-sustaining element through your body:

* Stand with your feet shoulder-width apart and place your arms straight out in front of you.

* Slowly do a deep knee bend.

* Squeeze your buttocks on the way back up.

* Repeat 10 times.

Studies reveal that the more social connections you have, the better your overall health.

# Balance Your Energy Fields

Polarity therapy is a holistic approach to healing that aims to balance the body's energy systems. Negative thoughts, pain, tension, stress, and environmental factors contribute to restricted energy flow. Polarity therapy gently manipulates your muscles to unblock energy flow and rebalance your body.

# Hands-On Healing

*Reiki*, which means "universal life energy," is a Japanese healing therapy. The vital energy of the universe is channeled through the practitioner to remove energy blockages and revitalize your body on subtle levels that promote wholeness, harmony, and balance.

# ACU
# PRESSURE

Based on the theory of acupuncture,
acupressure stimulates special points
on the body to help relieve pain
and boost energy
without needles.

# Stimulating Herbal Bath

*This herbal bath will invigorate your skin as it rejuvenates your senses.*

> 1 cup fresh *or* ½ cup dried rosemary, lemon verbena, or sage
> 1 cup Epsom salts
> 2 teaspoons olive or sweet almond oil

**1.** Pour 1 quart of boiling water over the herbs, cover, and steep for 30 minutes. Strain and pour into the bathwater.

**2.** Add the Epsom salts and oil. Blend well.

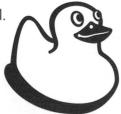

The more
challenging
the situation,
the more intrigued
you become.
Find something
challenging
to do today!

# Peppermint Pizzazz Tea

*Intensify the potency of your peppermint tea with this energizing zing.*

2 tbsp. fresh *or* 1 tbsp. dried peppermint
1–2 drops peppermint essential oil

**1.** Pour 1 cup of boiling water over the herbs. Cover and steep for 10 minutes. Strain.

**2.** Add the peppermint essential oil. Sip the tea slowly as you inhale the invigorating steam.

# Treat Your Feet

Wooden footsie rollers come in all shapes and sizes. Some are handheld, and others sit on the floor. The kind with raised ridges are both stimulating and relaxing. If you don't have a footsie roller, a wooden rolling pin can be used in a pinch. Simply place the footsie roller or rolling pin on the floor, bear down comfortably, and roll your entire foot back and forth. Repeat, concentrating on your arches for 5 to 10 minutes per foot.

"The people who **live long** are those **who long to live.**"

Anonymous

# Point and Flex

This is a great exercise to rev up the circulation in your legs and put the spring back in your step.

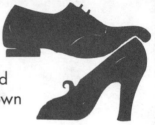

* Take your shoes off; sit on the floor with your legs stretched out in front of you and your palms facing down at your sides.

* Point your toes as hard as you can and hold for 5 seconds, then flex your feet as hard as you can and hold for 5 seconds.

* Repeat 10 times.

Did you know that something as simple as **boredom** can bring on **chronic fatigue?**

Try to exercise **OUTSIDE** to help oxygenate your cells with fresh air and facilitate the removal of waste products through your skin. Exercise improves cardiovascular fitness, endurance, and energy. If you live in a city, try to find a park in which to exercise. If city streets, with their attendant pollution, are your only outdoor option, exercising in a gym may be a better alternative.

# SHELL FISH

Shrimp, scallops, clams, crab, abalone, lobster, snails, crayfish, oysters, conch, and prawns increase energy, ease tension, and stabilize moods. Eat two servings per week.

If you wake up feeling groggy and sluggish, begin your day with some gentle stretching exercises to get your blood and oxygen flowing.

# Lemon Lover's Lift

*This herbal tea blend will help recharge your mental powers.*

MAKES 2 CUPS

2 teaspoons dried lemon balm leaves
2 teaspoons dried lemon verbena leaves
2 teaspoons dried lemongrass

**1.** Pour 2 cups of boiling water over the herbs, cover, and steep for 5 to 10 minutes. Strain.

**2.** Add a squirt of fresh lemon juice, orange juice, honey, or maple syrup to taste.

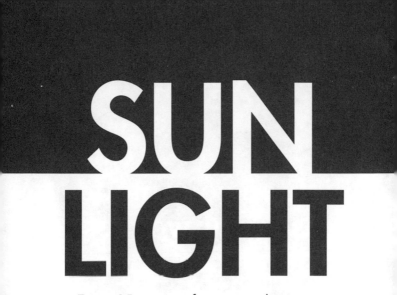

# SUN LIGHT

Ten to 15 minutes of unprotected exposure
to sunlight several times a week
is essential for healthy skin and bones.
Sun exposure also energizes your body.

A good heart-to-heart conversation can lighten your mood, ease your worries, and restore your connection to others.

# Toe Pulls

Try this simple massage technique when you're feeling frazzled. Hold your foot in one hand and grasp your big toe with the thumb and index finger of your other hand. Slowly and firmly pull on your toe, starting at the base and sliding your fingers to the top. Gently squeeze and roll the toe between your thumb and index finger. Repeat on the remaining toes, then switch feet.

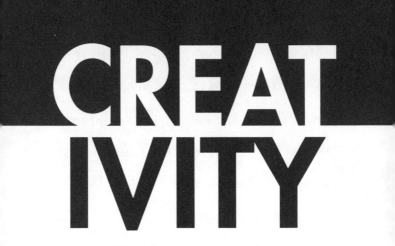

# CREATIVITY

Nourish your creative spirit.

Find creative ways to integrate family time with exercise. If you have children, don't just be a bystander at the **PLAYGROUND** — climb the jungle gym or play softball. Push a jogging stroller. Get a baby seat for your bicycle or sign up for swimming lessons together at the YMCA.

There's no better way to energize your body, mind, and spirit than by taking care of yourself.

"Never esteem anything of advantage to you that will make you break your word or lose your self-respect."

Marcus Aurelius Antoninus

For a cool, nutritious, energizing snack, try frozen seedless **GRAPES.** To prepare, pluck the grapes off the stems, place them on a cookie sheet with raised edges, and put them in the freezer for an hour. Eat immediately or store in a freezer bag for later.

# Get a Pet

Studies show that pet owners live healthier, happier, less stressful lives. Dogs will help you get more exercise. Pets make great companions and live-in psychotherapists, too.

# Meal in a Cup

*Fortify your mind and body
with this nutritious blend of vitamins,
minerals, carbohydrates, protein, and fiber.*

*MAKES 1 SERVING*

1 cup plain, low-fat yogurt or
   fortified soy yogurt
½ cup ripe fruit
¼ cup almonds, raisins, or granola
1 teaspoon honey or maple syrup
   (optional)

Combine all ingredients and blend well. Eat
immediately.

"Health is something we do for ourselves, not something that is done to us; a journey rather than a destination; a dynamic, holistic, and purposeful way of living."

Dr. Elliott Dacher

# BRAIN POWER

To boost your brain power,
eat high-protein snacks, such as peanut butter,
sesame butter, or cottage cheese.

Eat **FRESH,** whole, unprocessed foods. Avoid empty-calorie, chemical-laden junk foods. They do nothing but satisfy a temporary craving. Real food satisfies your soul and truly **NOURISHES** your body.

Maintain a **POSITIVE** attitude. Negativity affects your mood, job performance, physical appearance, and health. Your mood is **CONTAGIOUS** to those around you, too.

Stimulate your brain. Don't allow yourself to become bored with life.

# HYDRO THERAPY

To increase your energy,
shower in water that's approximately
body temperature for 2 to 3 minutes,
then lower the temperature to very cool
for 15 to 30 seconds. Repeat twice.

# Energizing Bath Oil

*This massage oil can be used when you need physical and mental stimulation.*

- 1 tablespoon grape-seed, hazelnut, jojoba, or sweet almond oil
- 2 drops each of eucalyptus, peppermint, and rosemary essential oils

Blend the ingredients. Add the oil to your bath while the tap is running or use as a massage oil after a bath or shower.

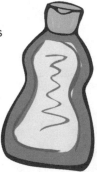

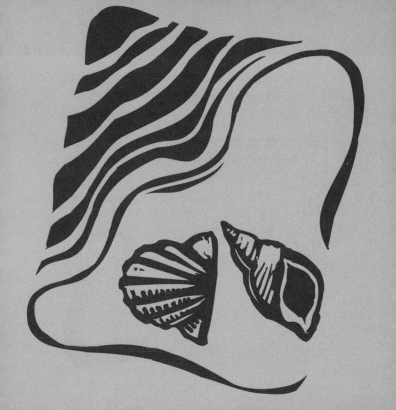

# Collect
# Memories

The next time you go on vacation, collect colorful seashells, stones, or other mementos. Fill an inexpensive, clear glass lamp base with your prize collection. You'll be reminded of your trip every time you turn on the lamp.

Nothing is more cheerful than colorful flowering plants. Select a few long-lasting and plentiful bloomers and put them in places where you spend the most time.

# Flower Power

Buy flowering bulbs for the dead of winter. Hyacinth, paper-white, daffodil, and tulip bulbs are perfect for "forcing." Insert the bulbs root-side down into an inch of white gravel, shells, or marbles in a shallow dish; add extra gravel to mid-bulb height. Set the pot in a bright, sunny window. Water with liquid flowering-plant fertilizer and keep moist until flowering is complete.

# INSPIR ATION

If your get-up-and-do-it
got up and took a hike a long time ago,
try listening to inspirational or
motivational tapes while you drive.

"I was always looking outside myself for strength and confidence but it comes from within. It is there all the time."

Anna Freud

# Learn to Cross-Country Ski

If you feel cooped up and lethargic in the winter, cross-country skiing is the perfect antidote. It's one of the best exercises for overall body toning, and your lungs get a work-out in the invigorating, chilly air.

For a **REJUVENATING** foot treatment, blend 6 drops of peppermint essential oil with 1 tablespoon of sweet almond oil. Massage your clean feet with the mixture for 15 minutes. Then put on socks to absorb the excess oil and condition your feet all day.

# Kick Off Your Shoes

Forgo the shoes and walk barefoot
in the grass. Let the warm, soft
earth caress your feet.

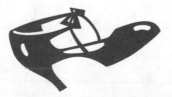

Whatever your passion in life, do it with gusto!

Many people think that **YOGA** is for people who can't do strenuous exercise. That assumption couldn't be further from the truth. Yoga strengthens and tones your muscles and joints by using your own body weight for resistance. It also builds **BALANCE,** coordination, and stamina.

# Give Your Body the Brush Off

For an invigorating morning ritual, try dry brushing to stimulate your circulation and shed your snake skin. Dry brushing is performed on dry skin — not oiled, not damp — but dry, before-you-shower skin. Use a natural-fiber brush to gently massage your body, except your face and breasts, for 5 to 10 minutes. Never scrub until you're red.

# Reflexology

This natural healing technique is based on the idea that there are **reflexes in your feet and hands** that correspond to your internal organs and body functions. Applying pressure with your thumbs and forefingers to certain points can relieve stress, improve circulation, and relax your mind.

# Reflexology Foot Massage

Try this foot massage to increase blood flow to your brain and enhance alertness.

* Hold the ball of your foot between your thumb (on the sole) and index fingers (on the top).

* Mentally draw four evenly spaced vertical lines from the tip to the base of your big toe.

* Make an inchwormlike walking motion with the outside edge of your thumb by bending the thumb repeatedly as you move it up and down your toe while applying pressure.

* "Walk" up and down each of the zones in your big toe designated by the vertical lines.

"Carpe diem —
seize the day."

Horace

# Enhance the Romance

Place several scented candles of varying heights in front of a mirror. Light them for a romantic effect. They will scent the air, and you can watch the flames flicker and dance.

Rediscover the joys of an imaginative journey through reading.
Keep a selection of soul-nourishing books at your bedside.

# Practice Deep Breathing

Enhance your energy level and ability to concentrate by practicing deep breathing.

* Close your eyes.

* Breathe in deeply through your nose and hold for a count of eight.

* Exhale completely through your mouth.

* Repeat ten times.

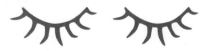

Communicate with nature. Explore the nearby woods, a garden, or just sit outside on the grass and appreciate the sights, sounds, and smells.

The lovely, floral fragrance of **LAVENDER** essential oil can soothe your soul without sapping your energy. To enhance concentration and promote mental clarity, place a drop on your wrist, the palms of your hands, or the nape of your neck and breathe deeply.

Do something
that will make you
feel good
about yourself;
buy yourself a
special treat or take
a day off from work
and do exactly what
you want.

# Self-Affirmations

Practice self-affirmations every day to keep a positive perspective. Here are some examples:

* I trust myself completely.

* I am a smart and talented go-getter.

* I am calm and relaxed no matter what the circumstances.

* I am at peace.

* I will not worry, no matter what comes my way today.

* I can do anything I set my mind to.

# Enjoy More Soy

Soybeans are touted as today's miracle food — and justifiably so. Abundant in fiber and complex carbohydrates, soybeans have an almost perfect amino acid profile, similar to that of animal protein. They even contain lysine, an amino acid not commonly found in many plant foods. Include tofu, soy protein powder, soy flour, soy nuggets, soybeans, and soy milk in your daily diet.

"The strongest principle of growth lies in human choice."

George Eliot

Sit quietly
and listen
to your heart;
it often gives
the best advice.

# PEANUT BUTTER

Incorporate this high-energy food
into your diet
for a perfect on-the-go snack.

# Clear Your Head

Take a day off and spend it antiquing, visiting a museum exhibit you've been longing to see, going to flea markets, or picnicking in a public garden. A change of scenery will do you good.

"Let no one
ever come to you
without leaving
better
and happier."

M O T H E R   T E R E S A

# RE
# CONNECT

Write a letter to a long-lost friend or relative.
Reconnect with loved ones.
Invest in fine, personalized stationery
and an exquisitely designed fountain pen
to create your own beautiful notes.

# Add Life to Your Tresses

*Stimulate your scalp as you add shine
and moisture to your hair.*

*MAKES 20 TREATMENTS*

4 tablespoons jojoba oil
1 tablespoon 80-proof vodka
2 teaspoons lavender essential oil
1 teaspoon basil essential oil
1 teaspoon geranium essential oil
1 teaspoon grapefruit essential oil
1 teaspoon lemon essential oil
1 teaspoon yarrow essential oil

Mix all ingredients together in a dark glass bottle. Shake well before use. Massage 1 teaspoon into your scalp with your fingertips for 3 minutes. Leave on for 1 hour or longer for maximum effect. Wash out with a mild shampoo. Repeat two or three times per week.

"A man becomes
what he
thinks about
all day long."

Ralph Waldo Emerson

# All-Day Energy

Eating several small meals rather than two or three large ones keeps your sugar level stable and prevents mood swings and headaches. It also regulates your appetite and ensures a steady stream of nutrients throughout the day. Digesting small meals requires less energy than large ones. Thanksgiving dinner makes you sleepy — remember?

Surprise
your loved one
with a special,
candlelit dinner
and a tempting
chocolate
dessert.

# Phone a Friend

Call someone who needs some cheering up. A bit of laughter and stimulating conversation will do you both good.

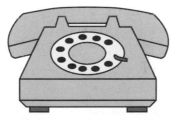

# Eat to Energize

Eat five to ten servings per day of the following fruits and vegetables. They're low in calories and high in energizing nutrients.

* **Berries:** Grapes, blackberries, blueberries, cranberries, strawberries, and boysenberries

* **Fruits:** Apples, apricots, peaches, bananas, pears, kiwis, grapefruits, lemons, oranges, and plums

* **Vegetables:** Loose-leaf and romaine lettuce, spinach, broccoli, Brussels sprouts, kale, carrots, tomatoes, red peppers, string beans, cabbage, onions, potatoes, and celery

* **Melons:** Cantaloupe, watermelon, honeydew, and Crenshaw

When you're feeling fatigued, try a short nap for about 30 minutes. Don't fall asleep; simply close your eyes and rest. This brief time of stillness rejuvenates your mind and body.

There is an old adage that "one must say goodbye before one says hello."

# LETTING GO

is an act of strength and courage. It helps healing begin, frees you of the weight of the past, and opens doors to a new future.

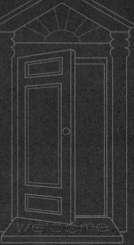

Be the kind
of **friend**
who lends
**a helping**
hand.

# Avoid Processed Foods

Reduce or eliminate high-fat dairy products, red meat, refined flour, and sugary foods from your diet. They sap your energy and increase your risk of developing cancer, arthritis, osteoporosis, heart disease, bowel problems, high blood pressure, and diabetes. Eat a wide variety of whole foods in as close to their natural state as possible. Unprocessed foods generally contain more nutrients, are void of questionable additives, and cost less than their processed peers.

Upbeat, **OPTIMISTIC** people are more likely to be healthy, energetic, and successful. A Swedish study of senior citizens found that mental health was an even stronger predictor of **LONGEVITY** than was physical health.

# Revitalize Your Eyes

Add two or three drops of calendula essential oil to a small jar of chilled eye cream. The resulting bright orange cream will help offset the blue color of dark circles under your eyes. Calendula is guaranteed to soothe and refresh tired eyes.

"Let's be grateful for those who give us happiness; they are the charming gardeners who make our soul bloom."

Marcel Proust

# Touch Therapy

The benefits go both ways. Touching another person exchanges healing energy, which results in a greater sense of well-being for both people. Research shows that hospital and nursing home patients experience quicker recovery when receiving touch therapy.

Strengthen the bond with your loved one by creating more intimacy together.

# Power-Packed Vegetarian Soup

*This delicious soup is rich in antioxidants, minerals,
and fiber and packs a nutritional wallop.*

*MAKES 6 QUARTS*

1½  quarts low-sodium vegetable juice
 5  cups water or vegetable stock
3½  cups crushed tomatoes
 1  package dried onion soup mix
12  cloves garlic, peeled
 8  stalks celery, chopped into 2-inch pieces
 4  medium white onions, peeled and quartered
 1  medium green cabbage, chopped into
    2-inch chunks
 1  large green pepper, chopped into 2-inch
    chunks
 1  habanero pepper, stem and seeds removed
 1  large red pepper, chopped into 2-inch
    chunks

1. In a 6-quart stockpot, heat the vegetable juice, water or vegetable stock, crushed tomatoes, and onion soup mix.

2. Grind the garlic, celery, onion, cabbage, and peppers in batches in a food processor until almost minced. Add to soup stock. Mix well.

3. Cover, reduce the heat to a simmer, and cook for 2 hours, stirring occasionally.

# You Are What You Drink

Try to avoid coffee, black tea, soda, alcohol, and refined juices. Coffee and black tea are addictive stimulants. They stain your teeth and leave you dehydrated. Soda is loaded with chemicals and phosphoric acid, which decays tooth enamel and leaches calcium from your bones. Alcohol damages your liver and kidneys and acts as a powerful diuretic. The excessive processing of refined juices removes their life force.

# SNACK TIME

For a healthful, nutrient-dense snack,
grab a handful of raw walnuts or Brazil nuts,
or chop them and add them to your salads
in lieu of croutons.

Life's best lessons
are learned from
life's problems —
these are your
teachers.

# Shovel Some Snow

If you're a northerner, throw away your snow blower and pick up a shovel. The lunging, lifting, and heaving deliver an intense workout, and shoveling gets you outdoors, too. You may even develop an appreciation for the beauty of snow.

# Mow Your Lawn

Get in shape and save money by mowing your lawn yourself. Using a push mower rather than a power mower provides all-over body conditioning.

"The best way
to predict
your future
is to create it."

Peter Drucker

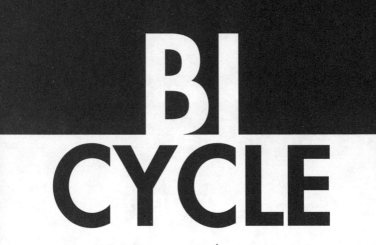

# BICYCLE

Leave your car in the garage
and dust off that old bike. Use it for
all your short errands instead of driving.

# Make Lunchtime Work for You

Use your lunchtime to go outside, breathe deeply, and move your body. It's a terrific way to recharge yourself so you'll be at your peak productivity level in the afternoon.

Buy a book of **AFFIRMA-TIONS** and carry it with you. Read it throughout the day to lift your spirits and instill confidence.

# Conscious Breathing

We are a society of shallow, tidal breathers. Constantly rushing around in a frenzy, we rarely utilize our full lung capacity, resulting in a constant state of fatigue. Most of us breathe from the upper portion of our lungs without expanding our diaphragm and taking a really deep, energizing and oxygenating breath. Be aware of your breathing habits and try to focus on breathing properly, which will energize your body and mind.

"**Without this**
playing with
fantasy **no creative
work has ever yet**
come to birth."

CARL GUSTAV JUNG

# VISUAL IZATION

Create scenes in your mind of happiness, health, and success. Fill in the details with sounds, colors, and scents. Pull up these images whenever you need a boost.

Look **FORWARD** to something. Plan a vacation, getaway weekend, or fun day trip. When stress strikes, recall the event you've planned for the near future.

# Kick Up Your Legs

You don't have to be a Las Vegas showgirl to have long, lean legs and tight buttocks. Place one hand on a sturdy chair, stand straight and tall, and kick your right leg as high as you possibly can without slouching or bending at the waist. Do 10 kicks, then change legs. Work up to 100 kicks per leg daily. This is a great cardiovascular exercise that jump-starts your energy, as well.

Wear red, orange, or yellow to brighten your mood.

# Eucalyptus Inhalation

*Eucalyptus essential oil has a camphorlike aroma that stimulates mental function.*

4 cups water
6 drops eucalyptus oil

**1.** Boil the water, remove it from the heat, and add the oil.

**2.** Drape a towel over your head and the pot and inhale the vapors for 10 minutes. Be sure to keep your eyes closed.

Be the kind
of friend
who laughs
at all jokes,
even if they're
not that funny.

Train for a local 5k or 10k fun run or benefit walk in your community. You may not break any speed records, but it will feel great to **ACCOMPLISH** a goal and to be among others who have done the same.

"You ask me
what I came into
the world to do.
I came
to live out loud."

Emile Zola

# Rev Up Your Posterior Circulation

Does your job require that you sit down all day? Feel like your fanny is spreading? Then learn to do isometric squeezes to stimulate circulation in your lower half. These can be performed anywhere, and no one else will know you're doing them. Squeeze your buttocks as hard as you can, hold for 5 seconds, and release. Repeat as many times as you can as often as possible.

# Flaxseed Oil — the Feel-Good Fat

Flaxseed oil is high in omega-3 fatty acids, which help fight fatigue, dry skin, itchy scalp, dandruff, arthritis pain, allergies, immune deficiencies, and constipation while improving eyesight and color perception. Consume 2 tablespoons daily. Ground flaxseeds are good sprinkled over salads, too.

# Stimulating Ginger Tea

*Ginger tea is recommended for flagging energy, colds, flu, motion sickness, and gas pain.*

1. Pour 1 cup of boiling water over ½ ounce of grated, fresh gingerroot.

2. Cover and steep for 15 minutes.

3. Strain and add honey and lemon juice for a unique, natural "ginger ale" taste.

# Blue-Green Algae

Rich in omega-6 fatty acids, beta-carotene,
and trace minerals, blue-green algae combats
fatigue, arthritis, psoriasis,
acne, and eczema. Take
2 teaspoons daily.

"You just can't beat the person who never gives up."

George "Babe" Ruth

Learn
to listen
to the messages
your body
gives you.

# Carbohydrates

Carbohydrates, organic compounds that furnish a large percentage of energy, are needed in a healthy diet. Foods high in carbohydrates include beans, fruits, rice, whole grain cereals, pasta, corn, potatoes, and bread. During digestion, carbohydrates are broken down into energy-producing compounds.

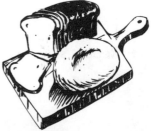

# A Gentle Awakening

Here are two yoga postures that are perfect for easing into your day.

* Start on all fours in the "table" position.

* Inhale, raise your head, and gently arch your back as you push your tailbone up into the "cat" position.

* Exhale, round your spine, push your hands into the floor, roll your tailbone down, and pull in your belly.

* Repeat several times.

Splash cold water on your face and run your hands and wrists under the cold water tap.

For a quick shot of **ENERGY**, stand up and do this exercise: Bend over at the waist and hang your head down so that your hands are touching your toes (if possible) and you're looking at your knees. Relax your upper body. Hold this position for several seconds, then slowly rise.

# Get Rid of Clutter

Lighten your load. Unclutter your closet, purse, office, bureau, garage, attic, and basement. Hold a tag sale or take everything to a local charity.

Tag Sale

"Life is a **daring adventure** or nothing."

Helen Keller

# Know Your Limits

Learn to say "no" more often to demanding friends, family, and co-workers who seem to sap every ounce of energy you have to spare.

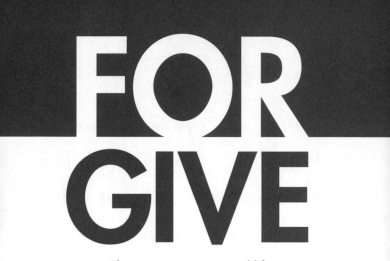

# FOR GIVE

Clean up your emotional life
by forgiving someone
who has done you wrong.

Call a good
massage therapist
and book a
full-body massage.
Your mind, body,
and spirit
will be completely
revitalized.

# Brewer's Yeast Mask

*This mask is recommended for those with normal to oily skin. It helps chase away a pasty winter complexion and removes dull, dry skin buildup.*

*MAKES 1 TREATMENT*

1 tablespoon brewer's yeast
1 tablespoon milk or water

**1.** Combine the ingredients to form a smooth paste. You may need more or less liquid, depending on the brand of yeast you use.

**2.** Spread it onto your clean face in a thin layer.

**3.** Let the paste dry, then rinse with cool water.

This mask may tingle as it dries. This is normal. If it starts to sting, rinse it off immediately and apply a good moisturizer.

# Enjoy the Little Pleasures

Are you so busy that you overlook life's little pleasures? Living at breakneck speed puts you on a wild roller coaster ride and makes you feel physically exhausted and spiritually frazzled. Set aside time for yourself, on a regular basis, to revel in the small, daily pleasures.

Poor **POSTURE** is hard on your spine. It compresses your lungs, depriving your body of oxygen, and accelerates gravity's effects on your facial contours. To improve your posture, walk around your living room with a book balanced on top of your head. Learn to adopt this posture.

# Boost Your Metabolism

Raise your metabolic rate — the rate at which you burn calories. Spices such as cardamom, ginger, cinnamon, onions, chili pepper, black pepper, garlic, and hot mustard help your body burn calories faster by producing internal heat. As a bonus, spicy foods stimulate circulation.

# Indulge Your Chocolate Craving

Chocolate increases the levels of the mood-boosting hormones dopamine and serotonin in your brain and is a source of phenylethylamine, an anti-depressant. Chocolate tastes great, too, so eating it stimulates the pleasure centers in your brain.

Get rid of
so-called "friends"
who are negative
or who bring
you down.

" . . . If one advances confidently in the direction of his dreams, and endeavors to live the life which he has imagined, he will meet with a success unexpected in common hours."

Henry David Thoreau

# Refresh Your Senses

Scented geraniums come in many fragrant varieties, such as rose, mint, spicy ginger, cinnamon, lemon, orange, peach, and strawberry. Put one on your desk or bedside table near a sunny window and gently rub the leaves between your fingers when you need a lift.

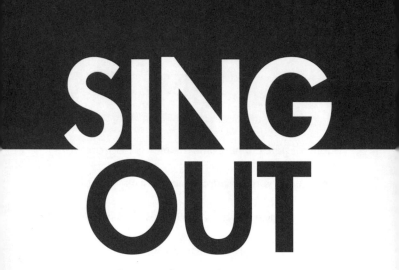

# SING OUT

Singing draws more oxygen
into your body, enhances mental clarity,
and banishes fatigue.

Your feet are actually more sensitive and **RECEPTIVE** to touch than your hands, because they contain a wealth of nerve endings. Sit on the edge of the tub and alternately blast them with cold and hot water at 10-second intervals.

Store your astringent or toner in the refrigerator. After cleansing your face, enjoy an invigorating rinse by **SPLASHING** cool toner over your face and chest. Your pores will look temporarily smaller and your complexion more refined.

# Rosemary for Remembrance

This pungently fragrant culinary and medicinal herb is a universal favorite for **boosting memory and mental performance**. Rosemary is available in the forms of essential oil, capsules, tincture, or loose-leaf tea and may also be used fresh or dried in your favorite dishes.

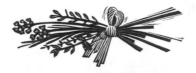

# What's So Funny?

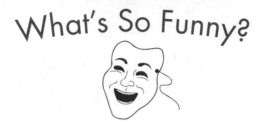

Laughter makes you feel good, makes your skin glow, and stimulates circulation and oxygen throughout your body. It also "massages" your internal organs. Go see a funny movie, read an amusing book, tickle your children, or play with your pet.

"Every day
is a birthday;
every moment of it
is new to us;
we are born again,
renewed for fresh
work and endeavor."

Issac Watts

# GINKGO BILOBA

This popular supplement
boosts circulation to the brain,
enhancing memory and alertness.

# Alternate Nostril Breathing

Try this yogic breathing technique when you need a quick energy boost.

* Sit down and close your eyes.

* Press your finger over your right nostril and inhale deeply and slowly through your left nostril. Exhale through your mouth.

* Press your finger over your left nostril and repeat the procedure.

* Alternate breathing through each nostril five times.

Green leafy vegetables, such as collard greens and spinach, are packed with folate, vitamins A and C, magnesium, potassium, and calcium. Eat a cup or more per week.

# Keep a Journal

. . . or a memory book. It's a great way to download the day's activities, reflect on the decisions you've made, and ponder the future. It's a soul-enriching experience to go back and relive your life's journey.

# Take a Hike

. . . or a walk. March in place.
Climb some stairs. Jump rope.
Do a few squats or high
kicks. Aerobic exercise,
even for just 5 minutes,
increases your energy level.

"Cheerfulness
and content
are great beautifiers
and are famous
preservers of
youthful looks."

Charles Dickens

Research has shown that people who eat **BREAKFAST** have higher metabolic rates than people who skip this vitally important meal.

"Develop interest in
life as you see it;
in people, things,
literature, music —
the world is so rich,
simply throbbing
with rich treasures,
beautiful souls and
interesting people."

Henry Miller

Scatter
fun minibreaks
into your
daily routine.

# Take a Dip

Go for a swim at the local YMCA, backyard pool, lake, or ocean. You'll feel powerful, graceful, and limber from this cooling energizer.

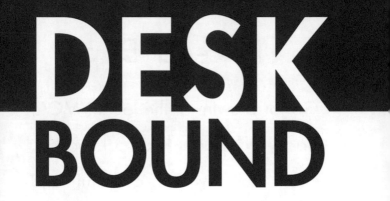

# DESK BOUND

If you're desk bound all day, try to get up
and walk around for a few minutes every hour.
Take the stairs at the other end of the building,
use the copy machine in another office,
or use the restroom on another floor.

# Embrace Yourself

Think about what makes you feel attractive, strong, smart, or energetic. Make a list.
Recite it to yourself when you need a boost.

# Share Your Artistry

Do you have a particular craft skill that might interest children? If so, volunteer to share your knowledge at a local camp, school, or library. Skills such as basic pottery, sculpting, drawing, painting, jewelry making, weaving, or basket making can be magical for children of all ages.

Value yourself
as much
as you expect
others
to value you.

# Beans, beans, the magical food

. . . the more you eat, the better your mood! It's true: Beans are high in B vitamins, which are mood stabilizers. They're also rich in complex carbohydrates, magnesium, iron, zinc, and fiber. A cup or so a day is recommended.

# Pick-Me-Up Tea

*Try this tea blend to start your morning
on an energetic note or to recharge
your stamina during the day.*

*MAKES 2 CUPS*

2 teaspoons dried ginger mint leaves
2 teaspoons dried orange mint leaves
2 teaspoons dried pineapple mint leaves

**1.** Pour 2 cups of boiling water over the herbs,
cover, and steep for 5 to 10 minutes. Strain.

**2.** Add a squirt of lemon or orange juice and
sweetener, if desired.

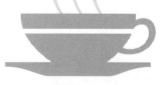

"Most of us will miss out on life's big prizes: the Pulitzers, the Heismans, the Oscars. But we're all eligible for a pat on the back, a kiss on the cheek, a thumbs-up sign!"

Barbara Johnson

Cultivate close
friendships
and renew old ones.
They can be
a source of strength
when times
are rough.

Your internal clock thrives on **CONSISTENCY,** so if you spend your weekends staying up late and sleeping in the next morning, your body perceives this as pseudo jet lag without even setting foot in the airport. Try to establish a regular routine and don't stray from it by more than 30 minutes to an hour.

# Herbal Body Wash

½ cup dried lemon verbena leaves
½ cup uncooked oatmeal
1 small muslin bag

Put the lemon verbena and oatmeal in the muslin bag. Moisten the bag thoroughly with water and rub it over your skin as a moisturizing pick-me-up. These small, fragrant bags also make lovely gifts.

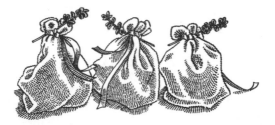

Make a list
of the past successes
in your life.
By remembering
your accomplishments,
you'll have the
confidence necessary
to achieve
even greater ones.

Decide what you want for your **FUTURE.** Stake your claim. Having a goal or vision will give your life direction, purpose, and passion.

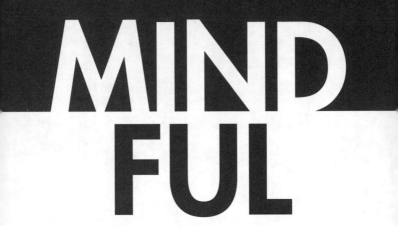

# MIND
# FUL

The act of being mindful
opens you to the full experience of the moment.

"Mindfulness provides a simple but powerful route for getting ourselves unstuck, back in touch with our own wisdom and vitality."

Jon Kabat-Zinn

Every
**big change**
begins with
**a baby step.**

"Affirmation of life is the spiritual act by which man ceases to live unreflectively and begins to devote himself to his life with reverence in order to raise it to its true value."

Albert Schweitzer

What we **MANIFEST** in this life is a reflection of what dwells deep inside us: our values, beliefs, and self-esteem. If we want to renew our lives, we have to change our inner beliefs about our right to happiness and vitality.

# Expand Your Horizons

Today, do one thing that you've really wanted to do but were afraid to try. Perhaps you've felt too intimidated or too old. Stretch yourself beyond your usual limits.

Paint the walls
of a room
a vibrant color.
It will lift your
mood every time
you enter
the room.

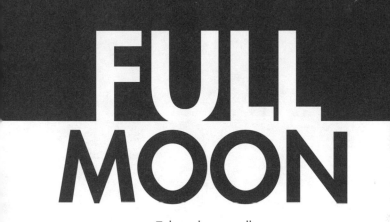

# FULL MOON

Take a long walk
in the light of the full moon.
Its quiet illumination
will balance your energy.

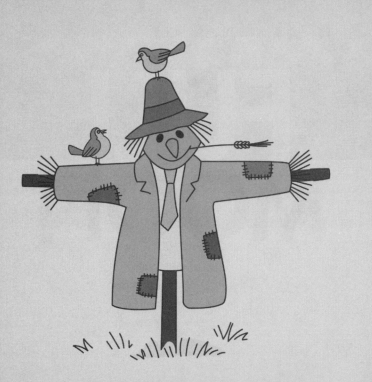

# "One who plants a garden, plants happiness."

Anonymous

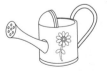

# Spice Up Your Day

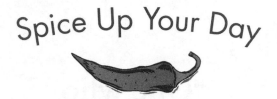

Cook a spicy meal for breakfast. Add hot salsa to your scrambled eggs, jalapeño jelly to your toast, or a little cayenne, cinnamon, and nutmeg to your oatmeal. Spicy foods stimulate your metabolism and awaken your senses for the day ahead.

Cultivate
an **attitude**
of **gratitude.**

"Happiness lies
in the fulfillment of
the spirit through
the body."

Cyril Connolly

"Many persons have a wrong idea of what constitutes real happiness. It is not obtained through self-gratification, but through fidelity to a worthy purpose."

Helen Keller

# What Do You Really Want?

Ask yourself with gentleness and patience, "In my heart of hearts, what do I truly want?" Be still, listen, and honor the answers that come. It may be a while before you hear the truest answer, which often speaks in a very quiet, almost imperceptible voice. This answer may be different from the life you are leading. That's okay. Simply live with this new insight and follow where it beckons.

Want to increase your self-esteem and personal pride? Develop self-mastery and uncover your hidden talents.

**PURSUE** only those things in life that support harmony, balance, inspiration, and spiritual enlightenment.

"Whether you think you can, or think you can't, you're probably right."

Henry Ford

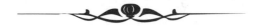

Put on your favorite rock 'n roll tunes, crank up the volume, and get up and dance.

Allow
your experiences
— good and bad —
to nourish your
spirit and give
you strength.

In our modern, hectic society, personal time is frequently shoved aside in an effort to accomplish more at an increasingly frenetic pace. **RECLAIM** your personal time and you'll naturally reclaim your own energy.

"Anyone who is truly concerned for the spiritual growth of another knows, consciously or instinctively, that he or she can significantly foster that growth only through a relationship of constancy."

M. Scott Peck

# Networking

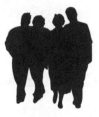

Build a supportive network of positive, affirming people.

# Ruby

Known as the stone of nobility, the blood-red ruby is said to gather and amplify energy while promoting and stimulating mental concentration.

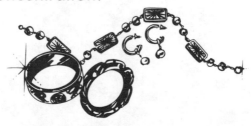

"This above all —
to thine own self
be true."

William Shakespeare

# Drink Your Greens

Green grasses, such as barley, alfalfa, and wheat-grass, and algae, including spirulina and chlorella, are touted as "superfoods" because they are chock-full of vitamins, minerals, enzymes, and chlorophyll. Available in health food stores in powders, capsules, or tablets that contain either single items or blends of grasses, algae, and herbs, these supplements provide quick energy and the long-lasting benefits of green vegetables.

"To so many people, goal setting means that only someday, after they've achieved something great, will they be able to enjoy life. There's a huge difference between achieving to be happy and happily achieving.

Instead of measuring your life's value by your progress toward a single goal, remember that the direction you're headed in is more important than temporary results."

Anthony Robbins

# Knowledge Is Power

Empower yourself by reading more books, watching movies, and attending plays. Visit museums, go to seminars, take classes. By expanding your scope of knowledge, you'll enlarge your mental reference library. This knowledge can be drawn on in the future — who knows where it could take you?

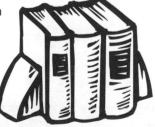

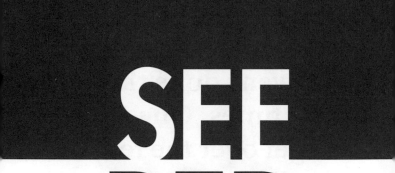

# SEE
# RED

Vibrant shades of red
have an energy-boosting,
highly stimulating effect on the body.

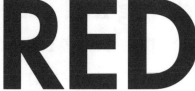

"Try a thing you haven't done three times. Once, to get over the fear of doing it. Twice, to learn how to do it. And a third time to figure out whether you like it or not."

Virgil Thomson

Add a little **ELECTRICITY** and variety to your life — attend a live, fast-paced auction, if only to listen to the auctioneer and observe the process. It's fun!

"Your soul
has designed
this life for you
in order for you
to learn its lessons.
Be grateful
for all those people
who have been your
teachers."

ROBIN NORWOOD

"Spiritual success comes by understanding the mystery of life; and by looking on all things cheerfully and courageously, realizing that events proceed according to a beautiful divine plan."

Paramahansa Yogananda

# Turn Down the Noise

Constant noise, whether it's from co-workers' conversations, machinery, traffic, or irritatingly loud music, can be stressful and physically exhausting. Try earplugs or a white-noise machine to drown out unwanted sounds with something more peaceful. Add weather stripping to your windows and doors; carpets also absorb sound.

# MentaliTea

*This tasty tea contains a special blend of herbs traditionally recognized to help restore mental awareness and vitality.*

*MAKES 3 CUPS*

1 teaspoon dried ginkgo
1 teaspoon dried gotu kola
1 teaspoon dried lemon balm
1 teaspoon dried nettles
1 teaspoon dried peppermint
1 teaspoon dried red clover

**1.** Pour 3 cups of boiling water over the herbs.

**2.** Cover and steep for 10 to 20 minutes.

**3.** Strain and chill. Serve over ice with a squeeze of lemon, orange, or lime juice and a teaspoon of honey, if desired.

See if you can still
do a handstand,
a cartwheel, or
a round-off.
It's fun to try — just
don't hurt yourself
in the process!

# Eat Healthy Portions

In an effort to control weight, many people, especially women, don't eat enough calories to sustain the energy levels necessary for everyday life. By eating less food than required for basic metabolic processes and normal activity, you run the risk of daily fatigue. If you're reasonably active and of average size, you need approximately 2,000 to 2,600 calories a day.

# Chyawanprash for Balanced Energy

What is chyawanprash? Derived from an ancient Indian recipe, chyawanprash is a dark brown, thick, sweet, and pungent paste of herbs and fruits. Available at health food stores, this special formula enhances vitality and strength.

The color **ORANGE** relieves fatigue and depression and enhances creativity. Wear orange clothing or look at something orange.

The color **GREEN** balances your energy. It reduces hyperactivity, yet helps eliminate fatigue. Focus your eyes on something green, preferably a beautiful lawn or woodland park.

"The good you do today may be quickly forgotten, but the impact of what you do will never disappear."

Anonymous

"Give me beauty
in the inward soul;
and may the
inner and the outer
be at one."

Plato

# Daily Energizing Drink

*This drink is rich in potassium, B vitamins, fructose, glucose, and trace minerals. Drink it twice a day, especially when you're feeling tired or suffering from stiff joints.*

*MAKES 1 CUP*

- 1 cup water
- 2 teaspoons raw, unheated, unfiltered apple cider vinegar
- 1 teaspoon raw honey

Combine the ingredients thoroughly and drink on an empty stomach.

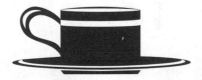

The color **VIOLET** is said to energize the brain. The color of royalty, violet stimulates self-confidence and joy.

"Enjoy life's 'puddles.'
Make cheerfulness,
outrageousness,
and playfulness
new priorities
for your life.
You can feel good
for no reason at all!"

Anthony Robbins

"Self-reverence, self-knowledge, self-control. These three alone lead life to sovereign power."

Alfred, Lord Tennyson

The color **MAGENTA,** a cross between hot pink and purple, is believed to raise energy levels. Try wearing this vibrant color as a wardrobe accent piece, such as a jacket, blouse, scarf, or pair of pants. However, an entire magenta outfit would be too visually overwhelming.

# Oriental Ginseng

*Panax ginseng* has been used in the Far East for centuries to stimulate energy and sharpen the mind. It's usually combined with other herbs in a tea or capsule blend, which gently and gradually strengthen the body's systems.

"Work
is love
made visible."

Kahlil
Gibran

According to nutritionists, **ZINC** helps increase endurance and prevents fatigue. Many people don't receive enough of this important mineral in their daily diets. Herring, oysters, meat, egg yolks, milk, and whole grains supply substantial amounts.

# Zippity-Do-Dah Juice

*This delicious fruit and vegetable juice
is rich in fiber, vitamins A and C, calcium,
potassium, and trace minerals.*

*MAKES 1 SERVING*

1 cup fresh pineapple
½ cup fresh dandelion greens
4 medium scrubbed, not peeled, carrots

Add all the ingredients to a juicer and drink
immediately. If the juice is too bitter, add more
pineapple or an apple.

"I went to the woods because I wished to live deliberately, to front only the essential facts of life, and see if I could not learn what it had to teach,

and not, when
I came to die,
discover that I had
not lived. I wanted
to live deep
and suck all the
marrow of life . . . "

Henry David Thoreau

# Shiatsu

In order to establish balance within the body, a practitioner of *Shiatsu*, a form of Japanese acupressure massage, applies pressure at strategic energy points on the body.

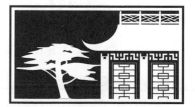

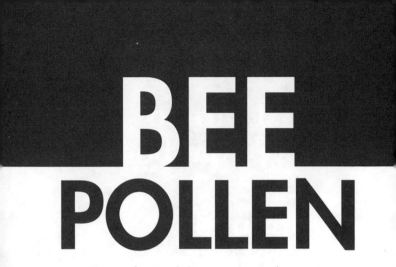

# BEE POLLEN

Known for its ability to promote longevity
and increase endurance,
bee pollen is available in granular form
from health food stores.

Learn to
love your body
in all its
strengths and
weaknesses.

# This Herb's for You

The lowly stinging nettle, *Urtica dioica*, a common pasture weed, is one of the best sources of plant-derived, highly digestible iron. This herb is also rich in vitamin A and calcium. Traditionally valued as a medicine as well as a food source, stinging nettle has been used to treat PMS, anemia, and fatigue. It's available in dried, capsule, or tincture form from health food stores.

# High-Energy Snack

Slice a large date in half, remove the pit, insert a raw pecan into each half, then sprinkle with coconut flakes. Make several of these little goodies, wrap individually, and keep them in your desk drawer at work, in your knapsack while hiking, or in your purse. They're the perfect snack to satisfy your sweet tooth and stave off junk food cravings.

"We confide in our strength, without boasting of it; we respect that of others, without fearing it."

Thomas Jefferson

Rose geranium essential oil relieves mental stress and fatigue. Inhale it straight from the bottle for quick **REVITALIZATION.**

# Help Others

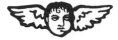

Visit local shut-ins and do a few things to show that you really care, such as taking out the garbage, watering the plants, going for a walk together, sitting outside, talking, listening, and holding hands. If your soul needs nourishment, find out how you can nourish others.

# A Mental Note

Did you know that staying physically fit as you age helps maintain mental fitness as well? It's a fact. You'll be better able to **learn new skills, remember things, and process new information.**

"What would you attempt to do if you knew you could not fail?"

Anonymous

# Treat yourself to a manicure.

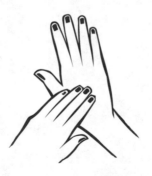

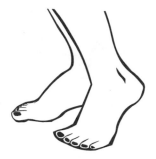

# Treat yourself to a
## pedicure.

# Hang a Bird Feeder

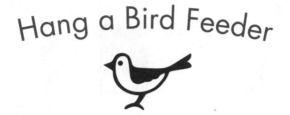

Hang a squirrel-proof bird feeder in front of a sunny window that you frequently pass during the day. Watch the birds that hang out there and remember to keep their supply of food plentiful.

"The love for
all living creatures
is the most
noble attribute."

Charles Darwin

Creating and **COOKING** a great meal can recharge your mind and body.

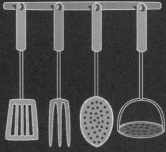

Eating what you've prepared is great, too! Even better is watching the faces and listening to the comments of friends and family as you dine and commune.

# Exercise for Endurance

Endurance activities, such as jogging, bicycling, swimming, and speed walking, combined with strength training, are the best exercises for boosting long-term energy levels. Aim for 45–60 minutes of exercise three to five times a week.

"Collaborate
with nature.
Value beauty.
Create an
environment that
entices fortune."

Victoria Moran

# Maximize Your Metabolism

Lifting weights enhances your metabolism. Don't worry, ladies — you won't get big, chunky muscles. You're not equipped with the necessary hormones. Try to fit it in two or three times a week.

# MOTI VATION

Break up exercise into 10-minute segments
and you'll feel more motivated
to fit several segments into your day.

# Energy from Housework?

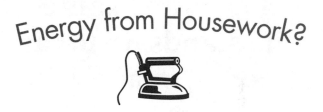

Believe it or not, **housework**, which includes washing floors and windows, vacuuming, cleaning your car, ironing, hanging clothes up to dry, and other drudgery, burns approximately 250 calories per hour **and energizes your body.**

"Each time some-one stands up for an ideal, or acts to improve the lot of others, or strikes out against injustice, they send forth a ripple of hope."

Robert F. Kennedy

Lemon essential oil has a clean, **INVIGORATING** scent. Add a few drops to your liquid cleanser or vacuum cleaner bag next time you clean your home or car.

"Even if it's a
little thing,
do something for
which you get
no pay
but the privilege
of doing it."

ALBERT SCHWEITZER

# Project Success

* Stand up straight and tall.

* Dress in flattering styles and colors.

* Walk as if you have someplace important to go.

* Take good care of yourself.

* Smile!

# Healthy Fats

A ready source of energy, healthy fats are one of three types of stamina-boosting foods in the diet. The most common fat-containing foods are cream, oily fish, butter, fatty meats, vegetable oils, eggs, nuts, and seeds. Try to consume 20–30 percent of your daily calories from healthy fats.

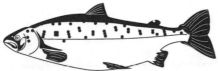

Seek out
the beauty
in your locale and
revel in it
as often
as possible.

"Faith is in many ways like a wheelbarrow. You have to put some real push behind it to make it work."

Anonymous

Smoking can cause fatigue
because it depletes the amount
of oxygen in your bloodstream.

Wild oat flower essence is great for when you're feeling aimless and uncertain about your direction in life. It strengthens determination, focus, and mental and **SPIRITUAL** vitality. Follow the label's directions.

# Turquoise

The blue-green turquoise stone is believed to protect the wearer from negative energy. Wear turquoise jewelry on days when you need spiritual strength and confidence.

# Good for the Sole

Fill two plastic foot tubs, one with hot water and one with cold water. Step from one to the other every 10 seconds. Dry your feet briskly by rubbing them with a coarse towel, and then slather them with your favorite cream.

To achieve a larger goal, start by implementing small, easily manageable steps.

# Zap Muscle Tension

If you sit or stand all day, your arms and shoulders can collect muscle tension. Try this exercise to release muscle fatigue:

* Stand up straight and raise your arms over your head as high as you can reach.

* Clasp your fingers together.

* Stretch and reach toward the sky.

* Slowly drop your head back, then forward.

"Think of the fierce energy concentrated in an acorn! You bury it in the ground, and it explodes into a giant oak!"

George Bernard Shaw

"Inside myself
is a place
where I live
all alone and that's
where you renew
your springs
that never dry up."

Pearl S. Buck

Feeling **NOSTALGIC?** Reread your high school yearbook, look through an old photo album, or sort through old letters. Reliving fun memories will give you a lift.

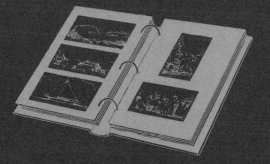

# Quick Spritz

Keep a spray bottle of cool water handy in your desk, briefcase, purse, or car. A quick spritz of cool water on your face will instantly revive your flagging energy and hydrate your skin.

# Let There Be Light

One of the easiest ways to boost your energy is with natural light. Open the curtains, lift the shades, add a few lamps with full-spectrum light bulbs, and let the sun shine in.

# Instant Energy

Drink a large glass of ice-cold water or tea. The cold fluid will shock your system into alertness.

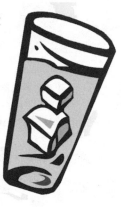

"There is something infinitely healing in the repeated refrains of nature — the assurance that dawn comes after night, and spring after the winter."

Rachel Carson

"The soul
should always
stand ajar,
ready to welcome
the ecstatic
experience."

Emily Dickinson

# Avoid
# High-Fat Meals

Fats stay in your stomach longer than protein or carbohydrates, leaving you feeling satisfied, yet diverting blood away from your muscles, brain, and tissues. Excess fat consumption can make you feel sluggish and unusually tired for 4 to 6 hours afterward.

The mind and heart need continued emotional and spiritual **GROWTH** and a fulfillment of dreams, goals, and desires. These are the foods on which our souls thrive.

"To love oneself
is the beginning
of a lifelong
romance."

Oscar Wilde

# Decorate Mealtime

Use bold, colorful place mats on the table with coordinating glasses and candles. A bright, cheery table will lift your mood every time you sit down for a meal.

"Always be
a first-rate version
of yourself,
instead of a
second-rate version
of somebody else."

Judy Garland

**REDECORATE** part of your house or apartment. Perhaps that stairway is too dim, or the hallway is long and boring, or your bedroom is too somber. Liven it up with paint, plants, pictures, or lights.

# Neroli Essential Oil

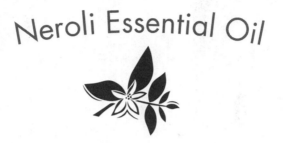

Derived from bitter-orange blossoms, neroli essential oil has a rich, intoxicating, floral fragrance that balances and uplifts the psyche. Place a few drops on a handkerchief and deeply inhale the aroma.

"When I go into my garden with a spade, and dig a bed, I feel such an exhilaration and health that I discover that I have been defrauding myself all this time in letting others do for me what I should have done with my own hands."

Ralph Waldo Emerson

# Listen to Your Body

If you eat when you're hungry and stop when you feel satisfied, you'll naturally have plenty of energy. But if you eat until you're stuffed and don't listen to your body's signals of fullness, your energy will wane.

# Revitalizing Room Spray

*For a refreshing, deodorizing,*
*mentally revitalizing room spray,*
*try this blend.*

½ cup distilled water
15 drops lemongrass essential oil
5 drops petitgrain essential oil

**1.** Combine the ingredients and add to a small spray bottle.

**2.** Shake well before each use.

**3.** Spray into the surrounding air.

# Juniper Berry Essential Oil

Juniper berry essential oil has a woodsy, refreshing aroma that men usually prefer to a more floral fragrance. It can be used for mental stimulation during times of stress and fatigue. Add 20 drops to ½ cup of distilled water and store in a spray bottle. Shake well before each use. This formula also doubles as a skin toner for oily skin and acne.

Add fuel to your furnace by consuming more **PUMPKIN.** It's not just for Thanksgiving anymore! This squash is so nutritious it should be eaten year-round in breads, soups, muffins, and casseroles. Pumpkin is rich in complex carbohydrates, vitamin A, fiber, iron, magnesium, and potassium.

"The man who has planted a garden feels that he has done something for the good of the whole world."

CHARLES DUDLEY WARNER

Take a music **APPRECIATION** course that focuses on your favorite type of music or, better yet, one that focuses on types of music of which you have limited knowledge. Remember: Music lifts the mortal soul.

# Lentil Soup

Just one cup of this hearty, energizing soup contains plenty of complex carbohydrates, protein, fiber, vitamins, and minerals and almost no fat. Many commercial brands are available — choose an organic variety with low sodium.

Watch the sunrise and absorb the oranges, yellows, pinks, and reds into your innermost being. These are the colors of fire, heat, and energy.

" . . . Creativity always means the doing of the unfamiliar, the breaking of new ground . . . "

Eleanor Roosevelt

According to modern physics, sound is kinetic energy, or energy in motion.

# Get Up and Go Perfume

*This light, refreshing perfume
will lift your spirits.*

2 teaspoons jojoba oil
4 drops bergamot essential oil
4 drops lemon essential oil
4 drops neroli essential oil
4 drops tangerine essential oil

Blend and store in a small,
dark bottle. Dab a drop on
each wrist, rub together, and
inhale the vapors.

**Note:** Do not apply to
sensitive skin.

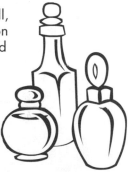

# Focus Your Energy and Creativity

Unclutter and organize your work area so you won't be distracted by the mess or by another project.

"Soul doesn't pour into life automatically. It requires our skill and attention."

Thomas Moore

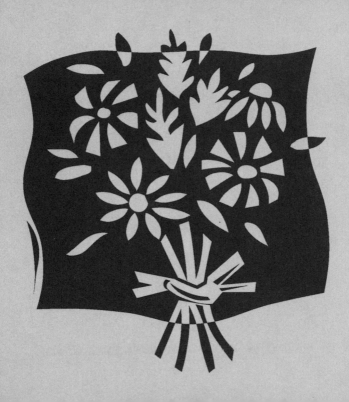

"If you take
a flower
in your hand
and really look at it,
it's your world
for the moment."

Georgia O'Keefe

# Sunflowers

The beautiful, golden sunflower, used as a survival food by the Native Americans, can still be consumed to increase physical energy and stamina. Boil the very young flower heads in water and eat them like Brussels sprouts or eat the seeds, either raw or toasted. Sunflower seeds contain as much as 55 percent readily digestible protein and a generous amount of healthy fat.

Make connections with your local **COMMUNITY** or a group, such as a bridge club, quilting circle, reading group, walking or running club, or local environmental preservation society. Connection with others instills a sense of belonging and enhances your well-being.

Drop "if only" from your vocabulary.

# Traditional Chinese Medicine

According to Traditional Chinese Medicine (TCM), qi, or life energy, is expressed in vastly different forms in animals, the human body, minerals, and plants, yet it unifies the physical, mental, and spiritual qualities of energy throughout the universe.

# Qi Gong

*Qi Gong* (pronounced chee gung) is an ancient Taoist healing system that is similar to yoga in that it emphasizes proper breathing and specific body movements to stimulate and direct the flow of qi, or life energy, throughout the body. The main objective of Qi Gong is to balance yin and yang energies. This discipline is practiced by the Chinese to develop specific powers and to maintain health by collecting vital energy in the solar plexus.

"Exuberance
is beauty."

William Blake

# Amethyst

The amethyst, a purple quartz crystal, is believed to transmit stability, invigoration, and strength.

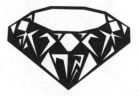

**GOLDENROD** flower essence repels negativity and promotes positive actions and thoughts. Follow the directions on the label.

"There can be
no joy of life
without
joy of work."

Thomas Aquinas

# Garnet

Considered the stone of health, the garnet, a dark red translucent stone, is believed to extract negative energy from the body's chakras, creating a more balanced state.

# The Seven Chakras

Chakras are energy centers situated in line with the spinal column. Subtle and unseen to the naked eye, the chakras absorb *prana,* or life force, from the atmosphere and distribute it throughout the body. The seven chakras are located on the crown of the head, brow, throat, heart, solar plexus, sacral section of the spine, and base of the spine.

**PENSTEMON** flower essence promotes inner fortitude. Follow the directions on the label.

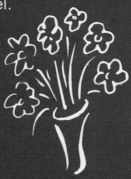

"The most beautiful thing we can experience is the mysterious. It is the source of all true art and science."

Albert Einstein

# Rhodochrosite

This striking pink stone with lacey, white patterns swirling throughout is believed to enhance spirituality and stimulate the vital energy of the body for optimal health.

"There is a
single magic,
a single power,
a single salvation, and
a single happiness,
and that is called
loving."

Herman Hesse

Find yourself getting bored with your usual fitness routine? Add **VARIETY** or change your scenery. If you normally exercise indoors, head outside. Try free weights instead of weight machines. Power yoga, Pilates exercises, or kickboxing can also recharge a stale routine.

# Magnet Therapy

Magnets attract and distribute balancing, healthful energy throughout the body. Healing magnets are available in different strengths and a variety of styles, including bracelets, necklaces, and shoe inserts. You can find them in stores that carry alternative healing supplies. Pregnant women and people with pacemakers, metal body parts, or metal pin inserts shouldn't use magnets.

# VitaliTea

*This strengthening and nutritious herbal tea blend enhances energy and well-being.*

MAKES 4 CUPS

1 teaspoon dried alfalfa
1 teaspoon dried horsetail
1 teaspoon dried lemon balm
1 teaspoon dried nettles
1 teaspoon dried oatstraw
1 teaspoon dried peppermint
1 teaspoon dried raspberry leaves
1 teaspoon dried red clover

**1.** Pour 4 cups of boiling water over the herbs, cover, and steep for 10–20 minutes.

**2.** Strain and add honey or lemon to taste.

**3.** Sip throughout the day, warm or iced.

"We know the power is available to each of us, every moment of every day, but we have to ask that the spiritual switch be turned on. Next, we've got to be ready to bear the Glory."

Sara Ban Breathnach

# Boost Your Qi

Methods for increasing the circulation of qi, or life energy, throughout your body and mind include yoga, dance, sports, moderate aerobic exercise, the martial arts, playing, and laughing. Breathing exercises and meditation also strengthen qi.

Share in someone else's **joyous moment and the happiness** will become **contagious.**

# Wear Copper

Copper bracelets help combat lethargy and passivity. Copper stimulates metabolism and is believed to bring good luck to those in its presence.

# Berry Picking

Simple pleasures can bring great rewards. Next time raspberries, blackberries, strawberries, blueberries, or huckleberries are in season, visit a local berry farm or friend with a backyard patch and pick a pail full of berries. Enjoy the visual feast of colors and textures.

"Whatever you believe you can do or dream you can, **begin it. Boldness has** genius, power, **and magic in it.**"

Anonymous

"We never know
how high we are
Till we are asked
to rise
And then, if we are
true to plan
Our statures touch
the skies."

Emily Dickinson

# Be Social

Do your favorite activities with a group whenever possible. A group of like-minded people acts as a support network, providing energy and motivation.

Create a **SPIRITUAL** path through daily meditation or prayer. Developing the often-neglected spiritual side of the human psyche can increase your energy and intuitive capacity.

# Art for Nonartists

Want to tap into your creative potential but have doubts about your artistic ability? Art has no rules; it is not black or white, right or wrong. Your artistic creations can be as abstract or as eccentric as you want. Art is the physical manifestation of your soul.

"When the mind is imaginative ... it takes to itself the faintest hints of life, it converts the very pulses of the air into revelations."

Henry James

# Kundalini

*Kundalini* is a Sanskrit term that means "spiritual energy in the body." When dormant, it resides in the first chakra at the base of the spine, where it remains ready to spring forth. The energy moves up the spine during the process of spiritual awakening.

# VOLUN TEER

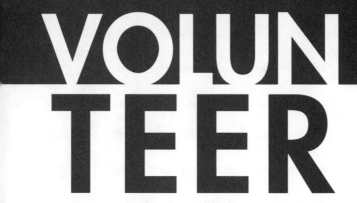

Your local homeless shelter needs you, and not just around the holidays. You'll get a spiritual boost by helping others and the realization that your current circumstances aren't so bad after all.

"Hope,
enthusiasm and
wisdom
are to the mind
as food
is to the body."

Dadi Janki

Want to stir the vital energy resting at your very core? Listen to a large choir during the holiday season or visit your city's symphony orchestra. This type of sound energy can affect your body and mind in **PROFOUND,** positive ways, creating balance, well-being, and motivation.

Read an inspiring
biography
of someone
you admire.

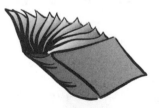

"Shoot
for the moon.
Even if you miss it
you will land
among the stars."

Les Brown

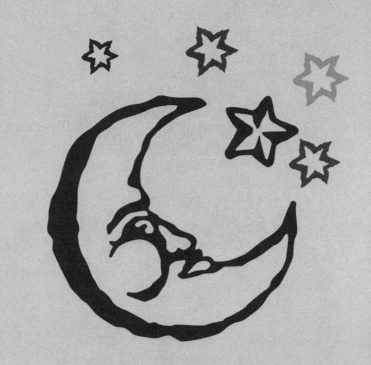

The yellow sapphire, yellow topaz, amber, and citrine stones are believed to increase energy and **VITALITY.**

# Bright Idea Tea

*Spur your creativity and mental awareness with this delicious herbal tea.*

MAKES 4 CUPS

1 teaspoon dried ginkgo
1 teaspoon dried hibiscus
1 teaspoon dried lavender
1 teaspoon dried lemon balm
1 teaspoon dried peppermint
1 teaspoon dried spearmint
1 teaspoon dried St.-John's-wort
Pinch stevia to taste

1. Pour 4 cups of boiling water over the herbs, cover, and steep for 10–20 minutes.

2. Strain and add honey or lemon to taste.

3. Sip throughout the day to keep your mood light and lively. It's particularly good on ice!

# Chanting in Its Simplest Form

Toning is a form of vocal meditation performed by chanting extended vowel sounds. Each vowel sound emits a different vibration, which can alter body chemistry and lead to emotional release, physical healing, and a heightened state of awareness.

"A friend
is a person
with whom I may
be sincere.
Before him,
I may think aloud."

Ralph Waldo Emerson

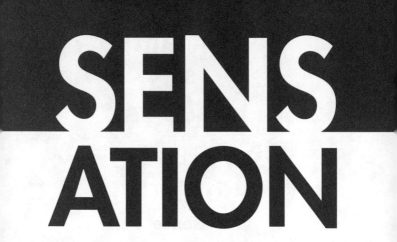

# SENS ATION

It's amazing how a simple touch can lift your spirits.
Ask a loved one to give you a hug,
hold your hand, brush your hair, rub your feet,
or massage your shoulders. Then return the favor.

# Flower Essences

These liquid extracts address the psychological and emotional aspects of wellness. Each essence holds the particular vibration or energy of the flower from which it is derived.

# Chant a Mantra

*Mantra,* a Sanskrit term that means "the thought that liberates and protects," is a sound used in meditation to balance the body and mind. A mantra can consist of a single syllable, a string of syllables, a word, or a phrase and can be repeated aloud or silently.

"Happiness is not a destination. It is the attitude with which you choose to travel."

Arit Desal

High in natural sugar, ripe **BANANAS** are storehouses of quick, healthy energy. They are a good source of potassium, magnesium, fiber, and vitamins B and C. Consume a few of these energy-boosting fruits each week.

# Unclutter Your Financial Life

Manage your money. Keep your personal and financial records in order to simplify budgeting and investing. Plan for your retirement, long-term housing needs, and financial requirements.

**IN-LINE SKATING** is a fun exercise for the whole family. Don't forget the helmets, knee pads, and elbow pads!

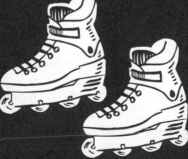

Don't wait for "the right moment" to start a new project — that moment may never come.

Be the kind
of friend
**who is supportive**
no matter
**what the**
**circumstances.**

"The shoe that fits one person pinches another; there is no recipe for living that suits all cases."

Carl Gustav Jung

# Take the Stairs

Avoid the elevator and take the stairs instead. It will get your blood pumping, and you'll get in a bit of exercise, too.

"If you've ever done any-thing successfully, you can do it again. Imagine and feel certain now about the emotions you deserve to have instead of waiting for them to spontaneously appear someday in the far distant future."

Anthony Robbins

"The human soul
needs actual beauty
more than bread."

D.H. Lawrence

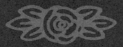

# Don't Worry

Worrying is unproductive and fills your mind with unnecessary, time-consuming thoughts. It limits your ability to enjoy life and be present in the moment. Focus your thoughts on things that bring you satisfaction instead.

# Food Allergies

Soy, dairy, wheat, corn, and eggs are the most common food allergens and can cause profound depression and lethargy in some people. If you're allergic to these foods, simply cutting them out of your diet can lift your mood.

"Each moment
and whatever
happens
thrills me
with joy . . . "

Walt Whitman

"We should consider every day lost in which we have not danced at least once."

Friedrich Nietzsche

# Tai Chi

*Tai Chi* (pronounced tie chee) is a martial art form that grew out of Qi Gong. It consists of a sequence of 100 or more movements performed in a slow, deliberate, ritualized manner, gently flowing from one motion to the next. It is a powerful form of exercise for toning the body while harmonizing the mind and body.

"The moon
has phases
from dark to full.
So do we."

Victoria Moran

Learn a new **CREATIVE** pursuit, such as quilting, gardening, cooking new types of food, or anything that will bring you lasting delight.

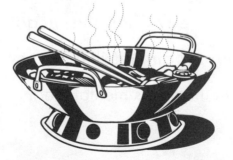

# Energy
# from Thunder

Take a walk outdoors after a thunder and lightning storm. Many people say that the negatively charged air resulting from the storm increases mental alertness.

"Falling in love
at first sight is as
final as it is swift . . .
but the growth of
true friendship
may be a
lifelong affair."

Sarah Orne Jewett

♥

"Every action that you perform is recorded in you, the soul. These imprints ultimately mold your character and destiny. When you understand this principle, you will pay more attention to bringing your best to everything you do."

Dadi Janki

# Dandelion Power

This lowly weed packs a wallop of nutritional benefits. Fresh dandelion leaves are loaded with calcium and vitamins A and C. Awaken a sluggish digestive system by eating the bitter leaves. Wild dandelions are a source of **energy and nutrition** offered by Mother Nature, free for the picking.

# Stay Focused

Focus on the daily moments of joy. Don't allow them to slip by unnoticed or ignored. Happy times provide an enormous source of power to your life.

Get
out of a
**dead-end**
career.

Visit a local cosmetology or hairdressing school for a makeover at a fraction of the price. Your fashionable, fresh **STYLE** will give you a new boost.

Learn a new skill,
pick up a hobby,
or take a class.

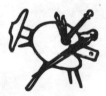

# Try to help someone every day.

# Chestnuts

The Iroquois, a North American Indian tribe, used to rely on the fresh nuts of the American chestnut tree as a food of great sustenance. The kernel consists of approximately 7 percent fat and 11 percent protein and contains energy-enhancing minerals, such as phosphorus, potassium, magnesium, and sulfur.

One of the basic causes of illness is unhappiness, and one of the greatest healers is joy.

Feeling stressed? Can't seem to concentrate? Balance your energy by listening to recordings of **NATURE** sounds, such as a crashing surf, jungle rhythms, or bird songs.

Wrap your arms
around yourself
and give yourself
a great big
bear hug —
you deserve it!

# Spread Loving Energy

Hug someone everyday. Energy has a rebound effect. When you give it, it returns to illuminate your body, mind, and spirit.

# Physiology Affects Psychology

Develop a physical habit of happiness. Depression often expresses itself in physical characteristics, such as a sad face, drooping shoulders, shallow breathing, and a shuffling gait. Make a conscious effort to stand up straight and extend a smile to everyone you meet. Intentionally making an effort to change your physiology will produce an uplifted emotional state.

You are **CREATIVE!** Can't seem to find the best way to express your creativity? Everyone is creative in one way or another, but perhaps you've lost touch with your artistic side over the years. Try to remember what used to excite you. What made your spirit soar? Rediscover the artist deep within.

# The Energy System

The human body is a dynamic energy system in a constant state of flux. We are an expression of the energy that permeates all living organisms and can be transferred from one organism to another. Just because you can't see it, doesn't mean it doesn't exist. In order for humans to survive, they must maintain a certain level of energy flow throughout their bodies. When this vital force ceases, we die.

Wake up and decide that today will be extraordinary!

# Other Storey Titles You Will Enjoy